SUCCESSFUL DASH DIET

AN EASY STEP BY STEP GUIDE TO LOSE OVERWEIGHT & REGAIN HEALTH

SUSAN MARGRET WIMMER

Made with ♥ on the Notion Press Platform
www.notionpress.com

Contents

1

Introduction

Obesity is a disease in which large amounts of fat in the body disturbs the functioning of most of the internal organs. This can lead to poor health. People with obesity are at high risk of developing a number of health problems: the higher the BMI, the greater the risk of certain diseases, such as heart disease, stroke, high blood pressure, type 2 diabetes, sleep apnea (cessation of breathing during sleep) and arthritis. The risk of cardiovascular disease increases sharply in women with larger waist and thighs. Weight gain in the waist (apple type) is more dangerous than weight gained around the hips and buttocks (pear type). Fat cells in the upper part of the body have a different quality than those in the hips or in thighs. The risk of developing diabetes, gallstones, hypertension, heart disease, stroke, and various types of cancer increases depending on whether a person is obese around the abdomen than on thigh or on legs. However, adults who are overweight and in middle age, face poor quality of life, as they age, and the quality of life is reduced as they increase the weight.

The major consequences of obesity are

Heart disease and stroke.

People, who are obese, have almost three times higher risk of cardiovascular disease compared to people with normal weight. As mentioned above, the weight concentrated at the abdomen and the upper part of the body most often associated with insulin resistance and diabetes, high blood pressure and unhealthy cholesterol and lipids. As a result, obesity causes danger to the cardiovascular system and results in ischemic heart disease, heart attacks and heart failure.

Insulin resistance and type 2 diabetes.

Most people with type 2 diabetes are overweight or obese, and weight loss may be the key to controlling the disease of type 2 diabetes. The common reason is insulin resistance - that is, the body cannot adequately respond to the insulin. This leads to an increase in blood sugar levels, which is a hallmark of diabetes. Insulin resistance is also associated with high blood pressure and abnormalities in blood clotting.

Metabolic syndrome.

Metabolic syndrome (also called syndrome X) is a pre-diabetic condition that is strongly associated with heart disease and high mortality.

Cancer.

Obesity is associated with an increased risk of developing cancer in general and some cancers, in particular. Studies have also shown that calorie restriction reduces the risk of cancer. Obesity can increase the risk of cancer; it is associated with high levels of hormones known as growth factors and can cause the rapid production of cells that leads to cancer. The researchers show many evidence on the link between obesity and different types of cancer as if endometrial cancer, breast cancer, prostate cancer and so on.

Joints.

Increasing amount of weight puts pressure on bones and joints. This can lead to osteoarthritis, a disease that causes pain and joint stiffness. In addition, people who are obese have a higher risk of carpal tunnel syndrome and other problems with the nerves in their wrists and hands.

Reproductive and hormonal problems. Infertility.

Abnormal body fat as high BMI may promote infertility in women and in men. Obesity especially connected with certain problems of infertility, such as uterine fibroids and menstrual irregularities. In men, obesity can contribute to reducing the level of testosterone and erectile dysfunction.

The effect on pregnancy.

Obesity has many dangerous consequences for the pregnancy. These include high blood pressure, gestational diabetes (diabetes, usually temporary, observed only during pregnancy), urinary tract infection, blood clots, prolonged labor, and a high fetal mortality rate in the later stages of pregnancy. Obesity is also associated with an increased likelihood of caesarean section. Children of obese women are also at higher risk for neurological disorders and birth defects that affect the brain or spinal cord, and other birth defects. Folic acid is generally effective in preventing these risks, but cannot be used as a protective agent in overweight women.

The effect on the lungs.

Obesity, especially moderate or severe, exposes a person at risk of hypoxia, a condition in which not enough oxygen to meet the body's needs. The intra-abdominal pressure, which results from abdominal obesity, pushes the diaphragm and compresses the lungs. These makes obese people put more effort to breathe. The lack of oxygen in turn causes chronic lethargy and ultimately, heart failure in the long run as a chronic reaction.

The effect on the liver.

Non-alcoholic liver steatosis. This condition can cause liver damage, similar to liver destruction in alcoholism. Steatosis occurs in half of all people with diabetes, and 20 - 50% of obese people, depending on the severity of obesity.

Gallstones.

The incidence of gallstone disease is much higher in obese women and men. The risk of stone formation is also high, when a person loses weight too quickly. People who are on the ultra-low-calorie diets, taking ursodeoxycholic acid can prevent the formation of gallstones.

Sleep disorders.

People who are obese tend to fall asleep faster and sleep longer during the day. At night, however, they needed more time to fall asleep, and they sleep less than people with normal weight. Studies have shown that obesity not only affects sleep, but sleep problems may actually contribute to obesity.

Sleep Apnea.

Obesity, especially apple type, is strongly associated with sleep apnea, when the upper throat relaxes and closes airway from time to time during sleep, temporarily blocking the passage of air. Sleep apnea is increasingly being seen as a potentially serious health problem that can lead to complications such as heart disease and stroke. Obstructive sleep apnea can also increase obesity. Some studies show that treatment of sleep apnea may help people lose abdominal fat.

Emotional and social problems. Depression.

Some studies have found an association between depression and obesity, particularly in obese women. There can be a number of factors that explain the link. People who are overweight may suffer from depression because of the social problems and low self-esteem. Usually, depression disappears when people lose weight. In men, the link between depression and obesity is slightly lower than that of women. Long-term studies have shown that women who are overweight are 20% less likely to be married, and 10% more problems with employment than their slender counterparts. However, studies have consistently shown that overweight men are not so much perceived emotionally as women of any age. Women and girls tend to blame themselves, while men tend to blame external factors for obesity.

2

Indicators of obesity in adults

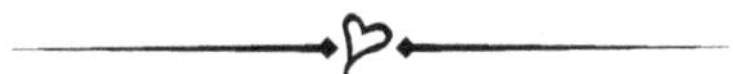

Obesity is the excess proportion of total body fat. Obesity is defined by measuring the body fat, not only by the body weight. One person may have a weight beyond the norm, but have a figure with a well-developed muscle and with low body fat. Another person may within normal weight, but an excessive amount of fat in the body.

The following measurements and indicators are used to determine whether a person is overweight to the extent that it threatens their health:

- Body mass index (BMI) - a measure of body fat
- Waist circumference (waist size)
- Waist ratio hips
- Skin fold measurements (anthropometry)

Body mass index (BMI)

BMI is an important component in determining health risks associated with obesity. Currently, one of the standards of diagnosing obesity is the body mass index (BMI).

BMI	Interpretation
Less than 16	Severe deficiency of weight
16-18.5	Underweight
18.5-25	Normal weight
25-30	Overweight or pre obese
30-34.9	Stage 1 Obesity
35-39.9	Stage 2 Obesity
40 and above	Stage 3 Obesity

These criteria may be used to assess the risk of developing complications of obesity, such as diabetes, heart disease, and certain cancers. They are also used to help decide when surgery may be appropriate.

The calculation of body mass index.

Body mass index (I) is calculated as follows:
Divide your weight m (kg) with the height h (in meters)
BMI is measured in kg / m2.

Waist Circumference

Waist circumference is another way to assess how much fat in the body. Extra weight near the middle part of abdomen increases the risk of type 2 diabetes, heart disease and stroke.

Some studies show that:

- Women whose waist more than 80 cm and men with a waist more than 94 cm have to watch their weight.
- Waist size of more than 89 cm for women and 102 cm in men is associated with a high risk of cardiovascular disease, diabetes and other complications.

The excess amount of fat in the abdomen (Increased waist size than normal range) causes heart problems and health risks than high degree of BMI.

Waist to hip ratio.

The ratio of the waist and hips. Fat distribution can be evaluated by dividing the waist size to hip size. The lower value of ratio shows better health status. The risk of cardiovascular disease increases sharply in women with a ratio of 0.8 or more, but for males, this ratio is above 1.0.

Anthropometry.

Anthropometry is the measurement of skin fold thickness in different areas, especially in the area of the triceps, shoulder blades and hips. This measurement is useful to determine whether the skin fold is made of a fat tissue or of a muscle tissue.

Statistics data on obesity

Over the past 40 years the number of people worldwide, who suffer from obesity, rose from 105 million in 1975 to 640 million today. If it goes on, in 2025 sufferers from obesity will be one-fifth of the world's population.

In recent years, the number of women suffering from obesity has increased three times, than men suffering from the disease, according to many studies. On the other hand, the probability that the WHO will be able to stop the growth of the disease in the next ten years is practically zero.

The need for change

The statistics and the consequence of obesity show that the obesity or overweight should be addressed seriously. How can you eliminate the threat of obesity? The most promising answer is DASH diet. DASH diet is developed to eradicate obesity and in turn, eliminates the complication, which arose from it.

You will be able to see further in this book about the ways in which the DASH diet eliminate obesity and its complications. In addition, you will get some idea on what to eat and what not, when you are in a DASH diet. This book will be your ultimate guide to reach your goal of weight loss with DASH diet.

3

DASH diet and Weight loss

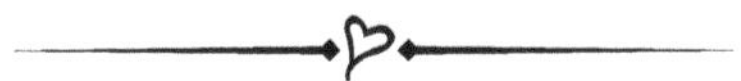

DASH-diet (Dietary Approaches to Stop Hypertension diet or to get rid of hypertension) over two decades ago, it was developed by American cardiologist and is based on a special diet with restriction of salt and sodium, sweets, sugar and sugar-containing beverages, fats and red meat. A major feature of DASH diet is to monitor, what exactly you fill your body throughout the day, rather than the quantity. Although those who aims to lose weight, it is necessary to monitor the calorie intake as well. In other words, the quality and the quantity of food that enters into our body is monitored in order to remove those excess calories and the complications which those extra calories caused.

The implementation of the DASH-diet uses food substances low in saturated fat, total fat and cholesterol, as well as plenty of fruits, vegetables and low-fat dairy products. That is, the daily diet must be sufficiently rich in magnesium, potassium, calcium, protein and fiber.

One of the main advantages of DASH diet is that it is not necessary to search for specific products and to develop culinary innovations. All that is needed is to analyze their own regular diet and adjust it accordingly. It will take about two weeks. As a rule, we have to add in more amounts of vegetables, fruits and grains (cereals) while reducing salt intake. The salt may be replaced with the use of spices, herbs or lemon juice.

If you are a meat-eaters, the portions of meat consumption also should be reduced to 200 grams per day. And be sure to include in your weekly menu for at least two vegetarian meals. It is a must to give an important place for vegetables and fruits in this diet.

There are no fixed DASH diet recipes, but you can make any of your own recipes into a DASH diet recipe by following these principles:

Create your individual diet DASH-diet can, using the following principles:

- Products from whole grains can make in your daily diet up to 8 servings. (Serving size - 1 slice of bread, 30 grams of dry cereal, or about half a glass of the cooked cereal, pasta, etc.)
- Low-fat dairy products should be taken 2-3 servings per day. These dairy products also serve as an important source of proteins. (One portion - 150 ml of milk or yoghurt or 40-50 g of cheese).
- Proteins from non-vegetables sources as if any lean meat, poultry, fish, eggs and so on. However, it should not exceed 200 g per day.
- If your daily diet contains no more than two vegetables, add another portion to lunch, and dinner. If your diet is little or no fruit at all - take them for snacking as an interesting alternative. In addition, the portion of oil, margarine and salad dressings should be halved, and

greater importance should be given to low-fat food substances. Moreover, the dairy products should be increased gradually. However, choose low-fat dairy products or, or non-fat dairy products.

- Fat intake should not exceed 3 servings per day. Portion - a teaspoon of vegetable oil or margarine, a tablespoon of mayonnaise, a tablespoon of the salad dressing and so on)
- Vegetables - 5 servings per day. (A serving - half a cup of vegetables other than greens, if green vegetables - then twice)
- Fruits - up to 5 servings per day. (One portion of fresh fruit is equal to 1 cup of fresh fruit, ¼ cup dried fruit or half a cup of fruit juice)
- The amount of fluid consumed, including a soup or fruit juice, should not exceed 2 liters per day. The fluid is one of the important parts of this diet. The fluid should be limited to 2 liters, but should not reduce than 2 liters per day. Too low fluid consumption can lead to dehydration.
- Low-fat sweets should be limited to 5 servings per week. (One portion is equal to one tablespoon of sugar or jam or a glass of soda)
- Nuts, seeds and legumes are limited to 5 servings per week. (A serving is equal to 40 grams of nuts, or 2 tablespoons of peanut butter or cooked peas / beans)
- The DASH diet is limited to 2000 calories per day. This calorie restriction is enough to achieve the necessary weight loss. In addition, the energy deficit produced by this DASH diet is enough to reduce 10-12 lbs per month. This type of calorie restriction can be managed for even lifetime, but it can be followed even for short period of time. However, this diet should be followed for at least 2 weeks in order to get positive result out of this diet.

Restrictions of Salt

An important part of the DASH diet is to restrict salt intake. On an average day, a person should consume no more than 2,300 milligrams of salt per day. This is approximately equal to 1 teaspoon of salt and is considered an optimum amount for an average person with no chronic diseases, as well as for middle-aged people.

However, the recommended amount of salt for people with hypertension, type 2 diabetes, chronic kidney disease, as well as for people over 51 years is 1500 mg of salt (3-4 g of salt) per day.

Moreover, it is very important to know that these 7g includes all of the salt we consumed during the day. However, many products available in the market are packed with salt and it is hidden most of the time. Nevertheless, it is your responsibility to sort out these products.

Products containing hidden salt:

- Canned food and canned soups
- Meat and fish products
- Sausages
- Chips, crackers, and popcorn
- Pickles and marinades
- Fast food
- Salted nuts, peanuts, snack
- Ketchup and sauces

It is very hard to achieve balance with these hidden salt-containing foods and salt less food in order to fit perfectly with DASH diet. Indeed, it is much easier to stop consuming all of the above products, than to suffer by counting salt amount in each of these products to adjust the diet. Rather, it is wise to focus on the ways to reduce the salt content in the food substance.

To reduce the intake of salt, use the following methods:

- Do not add salt to the cooking food at all. If you are cooking for a family, let each one of the members decides their salt intake and this makes the person who is in DASH diet to focus on his or her own salt intake. This is only a problem in the first couple of days. Later, most of us get acclimatised with this habit.
- Instead of salt, use spices, herbs, lemon juice. These substances are very sharp in taste and that makes these ingredients an alternative to salt.
- Instead of using canned products (canned meat, fish), take their fresh counterparts and cook them yourself.
- Instead of pickles, use more fresh vegetables or even use frozen vegetables in the summer as well as in the winter.
- Do not use frozen foods as if pizza, burgers, dumplings, nuggets, and so on, they are usually packed with a huge amount of salt.
- Instead of sausages, use real meat, but better to add chicken breast to the diet.
- If you are using Sauerkraut, you need to rinse them thoroughly to remove salt. It is true for most of the vegetables.

The table below gives us a rough idea on how herbs can be used as an alternative to salt:

Herbs

How they can be used

Basil

Soups, salads, vegetables, meat, fish, pasta, scrambled eggs

Carnation

Soups, salads, vegetables

Ginger

Soups, salads, vegetables, meat

Cinnamon

Salad, vegetables, bread, snack

Marjoram

Soups, salads, beef, fish, chicken, vegetables, scrambled eggs

Nutmeg

Vegetables, meat, appetizers, omelets, pasta

Oregano

Soups, salads, vegetables, meat, snacks, pasta

Chili (hot pepper)

Soups, salads, vegetables, meat, fish, sauces

Parsley

Salad, vegetables, fish, meat

Rosemary

Salad, vegetables, fish, meat

Thyme (thyme)

Salad, vegetables, fish, chicken

Caraway

Pilaf, rice, salads, vegetables

Dill

Soups, salads, vegetables, fish, poultry, burgers, shrimp

Sage

Soups, salads, vegetables, meat, poultry

The salt restriction does not alone facilitate the reduction of high blood pressure, but salt restriction has an important role in the reduction of weight. The salt is an important element, which retains water in the body. When the level of salt is high in the diet, the body tends to retain more water and results in weight gain. However, if the salt content is reduced, the body cannot retain water in the circulatory system of the body and results in the weight loss. It is very much important to keep the salt at its limit in order to achieve effective weight loss.

Restricting calories

The calories we consume should be managed properly, because the excess calories we consume are converted into fat by hormonal and enzymatic action by our body. This results in the accumulation of heap of fat in the body. This in long run leads to obesity.

However, DASH diet is based on 2000 calories per day. However, if you need to lose weight, you can limit the calorie intake to 1600 kcal per day. The calorie restriction in the DASH diet helps to reduce your total calorie needed for the day. However, what you need to do, in order to lose weight. The calorie spend should be greater than the calorie intake. This is the idea behind the weight loss in DASH diet. The calorie deficit should be created every day, so that the accumulation of these calorie deficit results in weight loss. Generally, you need to spend 3500 calories to burn 1 lbs of weight. This is the general rule to lose weight.

Moreover, the restricting calorie intake in DASH diet is supported by high amount of vegetables and fruits. Why it is important? Because most of them have negative calories. These are

- Broccoli,
- Cauliflower and cabbage,
- Tomatoes and cucumbers,

- Sweet and fragrant pepper,
- Black radish,
- Radish,
- Eggplant,
- Peas,
- Beetroot,
- Asparagus,
- Celery, parsley, spinach, basil, lettuce,
- Green bean,
- Zucchini,
- Onions (bulb and green),
- Garlic,
- Carrot,
- Grapes,
- Pineapple,
- Grapefruit,
- Peaches,
- Cherries and cherry,
- Apricots,
- Papaya,
- Melon,
- Mango,
- Kiwi,
- Pears and apples,
- Plums,
- Strawberries, blackberries, raspberries, blueberries, currants,
- Figs,
- Lemons, tangerines and oranges.

In addition, the calorie restriction is not done abruptly, but a gradual decrease in calories should be achieved through the following way.

Change your diet gradually

The diet change in a lifestyle is a very big step. You need to focus on how to amend these changes is the key to success. In addition, the change should be gradual rather than a abrupt change. Abrupt change always ends up in failure. Therefore, the introduction new food as well as reduction or elimination of food substances from the lifestyle should be happened in a gradual way.

Forgive yourself with diet violations

Everyone can make mistakes, especially when we begin to do something for the first time. Remember that changing your everyday habits is a long process. Therefore, you need to give some time. The cheat meals are all right occasionally, and those violations should be forgiven instead of making it a big issue out of the situation.

Reward yourself for success

Reward yourself with non-food prizes for achievements in the field of normalization of life.

Increase physical activity

To return your blood pressure to normal values in addition to compliance with the weight loss, you need to increase physical activity. Two simple changes in lifestyle - diet and physical activity - in their joint application is much more effective than each of them, taken separately, and is much more effective than medications. Recent research conducted by the American Heart Association, showed that those patients who had a clear motivation, able to normalize blood pressure and reduce individual risk of cardiovascular disease by changing lifestyle, by including the DASH diet and increased physical activity. All of these results are possible with DASH by its chief function of weight loss and it helps to stabilize the cardiovascular system.

Restriction of sweets

Sweets are very good in taste but are terribly bad to our health. Why do we say that? Sweets we consume are converted into glucose. The sweets we consume are generally packed with a huge amount of glucose within them. When we start to consume more sweets, the glucose level in the body goes high. This signals our pancreas to release a hormone named Insulin. Insulin is a hormone, which metabolizes glucose and helps to utilize this glucose by the body as energy. What is the bad news with the sweets? The extra high stimulation of pancreas can lead to an unresponsive status and thus the glucose is not monitored and controlled, due to heavy load on the pancreas. In addition, the unused and unwanted glucose in the body is converted into fat. This is the major way of the fat accumulation, which leads to obesity in very short span of time.

The restriction of sweets should be done in a gradual way; otherwise, the abrupt restrictions lead to increased sweets cravings. How do we do it?

1: Restriction of sweets as an initiation process

First of all, get ready for the fact that the rejection of sweet is a process but not a timely action. Timely restriction can lead to increased cravings throughout another day and you might consume all those sweets that you restricted for that specific period and more. However, restriction of sweets should be approached as a process by setting up alternatives to sweets gradually. You need to set a goal, so that you will need about a month to learn how to live in peace without the sugar, allowing the sweet from time to time and not falling down on overeating and regaining all of those sugars, which you avoided.

Remember that sugar is literally addictive - both physical and emotional. However, this addiction is not as bad as drug or alcohol addiction. But, you need to have a commitment in order to compromise with sugar restriction.

2: Avoid direct sources of sugar

The first step will be the non-sweet exclusion from the diet of foods containing sugar in its pure form - jams, carbonated beverages, packed fruit juices, chocolate and traditional sweets.

This fresh fruit and sources of fast carbohydrates (such as potatoes) to exclude from the diet is not required - it is important not to confuse with the restriction of sugar and carbohydrate-free diet. The sugar restriction is implemented to avoid the purest sugar that comes into our body. They are direct glucose and it can raise the blood sugar level immediately.

3: Fight the addiction

If in the early days of the refusal of sugar, you will feel that you are dying to eat something sweet, and all your thoughts are solely on this. You need to distract yourself with other facts of DASH diet. Increasing the intake of vegetables and fruits as in DASH diet helps to supplement sugary taste with the crunchy and sweet vegetables and fruits. In addition, these fruits and vegetables fill your stomach, so that your mind does not go to the sweets.

In these moments, you manage physical dependence of sugar on our body, so it is especially important to teach your body to work without readily available energy.

4: Avoid sugar substitutes

Fructose, which is a long time called dietary sugar substitute, proved to be even more harmful - in fact, the body converts its energy directly to fat deposits. The benefits of Stevia and other "natural" sweetener is also a big question.

Also, do not forget that you are opposed to the dependence with sugar, therefore, no need to once again remind our body about how do the sweets taste and this might backfire with sugar restrictions.

5: Remove sweets out of sight

An important step will be to audit domestic stocks for the content of sugar. Train yourself not to buy sweet "in reserve" and does not keep the sugar in its pure form at home. If you cannot drink tea without sugar, drink it with a drop of honey or Coffee with low-fat milk.

Replace cakes and other desserts with fruits and give up sugary breakfast cereals in favor of freshly squeezed fruits and vegetable juices.

6: Learn to see hidden sugar

The last step will be the abandonment of food containing a "hidden sugars" - that is, those products of the sugar content in which you had no idea. First of all, it is a variety of sauces and all of the fast foods or street foods.

Teach yourself to study the composition of the product on the packaging, as well as synonyms, which the manufacturers used to include for sugary substances as if fructose, fructose syrup, glucose syrup, glucose, dextrose, sucrose, agave nectar, and so on.

7: Change the attitude to sweet

Since it is practically impossible to completely abandon the products containing sugar or simple carbohydrates, it is important to learn how to relate to them as much as possible with the substances you have substituted as if fruits and vegetables. You need to understand that sugar in normal amount is not harmful, but if you use them in excess, it is a nightmare for your body.

Increased intake of Vegetables and fruits

DASH diet allows consuming more fruits and vegetables in order to lose weight. However, why vegetables and fruits? The fruits and vegetables should be consumed the most, next to carbohydrates. These fruits and vegetables supply us enough of vitamins, minerals, micronutrients and a lot of fiber. These nutritional elements help our body function properly. Minerals and vitamin B group participate in metabolic a chemical reaction, which takes place inside our cells, while vitamin C and E are great anti-oxidants. They deactivate and eliminate all the free radicals, which are byproducts of metabolic reactions. Further, the vitamins and minerals keep up our immunity, protects our skin, nails and hair. These elements are responsible for the beauty of our body outside as well as inside. The fibers from vegetables and fruits help the bowels form proper stools and evacuate the remnants of digestion in the proper manner. There are also soluble fibers, which help functions of the organs in our body.

Fruits and vegetables should be consumed five times a day. It is easy and it will make your meals more interesting. Just think, if you can add a banana for the morning cereal and a salad at lunch and boiled vegetables for dinner while two snacks a day with vegetable or fruit smoothies, you have taken all five. It is simple as that.

Fruits are everyone's favorite. Not only the colour and the flavor it has got, but also because of its nutritional value. All most all the fruits have a whole lot of Vitamins such as A.

B, C and D packed in them and then minerals too. Fruits are packed with potassium, zinc, magnesium, calcium, copper, manganese and selenium. These minerals are essential for our body's functions and its healthy balance. All the fruits are also packed with a whole lot of anti-oxidants and phyto-nutrients. These phyto-nutrients are micronutrients, which cannot be classified as minerals or vitamins, yet, plays a major role in keeping our body healthy.

The anti-oxidant content is very high in citrus than in any other fruit or vegetable. But, even the fruits contain a great amount of antioxidants in the form of vitamin C, flavonoids and anthocyanins. They help to remove the free radicals from our body. They fight against those components, which can damage our cells and make us sick. And also these antioxidants are good in stimulating our immunity and fighting against infections. Vitamin C also helps our body to absorb minerals, especially iron and we know that iron is a main element of our blood. To tell the truth, not only our blood, but many chemical reactions happening inside the cells of our body needs iron, magnesium, calcium and zinc.

How can these minerals and vitamins help us? Fruits have simple sugars, mostly in the form of fructose. They taste sweet, but, it is not by those refined sugars which we eat and which has become the enemy of our health in this modern world, but, it is a simple sugar called fructose. It is natural, tasty and also is healthy. Fructose is not sucrose to be converted to glucose; therefore, even diabetic patients can enjoy them.

Anthocyanins are flavonoids found in most of berries. When making infused waters using these fruits, these anthocyanins dissolve and add a light colour to the water. These pigments offer many health benefits. These compounds have potent antioxidant properties, which aids in the elimination of free radicals from our body, and thus offer protection against cancers, aging, infections, etc.

The next secret of fruits is that it gives us a glowing skin; A skin free of wrinkles, dryness and pigmentations. Thanks to all those microelements in fruits. They are above any facial kits, creams, gels and to tonics. Once they go down the throat, they reach our skin; concentrates there, resulting a soft, smooth glowing skin.

Vegetables also contain great amount of soluble fibers than the fruits. They are very useful in preventing rise in cholesterol level of the body and also if you are already in a diet plan, these waters may give a feeling of fullness to your stomach and delay your hunger.

Try adding three vegetables for each meal you consume and a fruit dessert to accompany the meal. After knowing the importance facts, are you going to tell any more that DASH diet only helps to lose weight?

4

Benefits of DASH diet Beyond Weight loss

DASH diet is initially designed to aid people who are suffering from Hypertension. The DASH diet restricts the amount of fluids and salt consumption. What happens to our body? The salt and the fluids have direct role in increasing the blood pressure. The increase intake of the salt can disturbs the balanced environment created by our kidney. Our kidney performs the elimination of waste substances from our body. They are also helping in balancing the fluid content as well as the minerals in our body. The increasing amount of certain minerals or ions can cause serious effect on the body, so the kidneys eliminate those elements from our body. However, increase in salt amount leads to change in the osmotic balance of our blood. This disturbs the balance created by the kidney. As a reaction to it, our body increases the function of kidneys to remove fluid from our body, but the increased salt content retains water. The net effect of the reaction is increased blood pressure. This increment in the pressure damages the kidneys and in long run can lead to kidney failure.

However, DASH diet restricts the amount of salt. When these two parameters are set in optimal level, the blood pressure comes back to normal range.

Another important fact that the DASH diet helps to reduce high blood pressure through weight loss. Obesity, especially abdominal obesity increases the blood pressure by 1-2 mm every few inches of increment of the waist size. However, the DASH diet addresses the problem of obesity and hence, indirectly reduces the high blood pressure.

In addition, the increased blood pressure exerts heavy pressure on our arteries. As a result, small arteries increase their wall strength by increasing its size. This reaction to high blood pressure makes the blood to flow through them with high resistant. All of these reactions increase the blood pressure again and as a result, the pressure of the blood goes level beyond our norm. But, the use of DASH diet, reverses these effects of the arteries due to hypertension and thus the major functions of the arteries as of supplying nutrients and oxygen to organ restore.

In addition, high blood pressure put our heart also at risk of developing angina. However, the pressure and the body fat reduce the risk of developing further cardiovascular diseases.

Moreover, the DASH diet is packed with high level of antioxidants. These antioxidants are coming from vegetables and fruits. These antioxidants act as a anti-ageing agent. The increased amount of free radicals in the body leads to activation of ageing process, but these antioxidants has the power to flush out the free radicals from the body and thus promote glowing skin.

In addition, antioxidants detoxify our body and prepare the body towards the new beginning with DASH diet. The detoxification property of the antioxidants also acts as a protector of our liver. This also protects the liver from developing severe stage of fatty liver disease due to increased cholesterol in the body as a result of obesity.

5

Pros and cons of the DASH-diet

PROS

i. It is completely safe for health.
v. It is recommended by most of the doctors and is not injurious to health.
v. It allows you to not only lose weight but also to improve overall health.
v. Do not have to feel a sense of hunger.
v. Foods that are recommended in the DASH diet are simple and accessible and it does not require any extra effort to keep the achieved results.
v. Food items that are needed in DASH diet do not cost more than the usual daily diet.
v. It does not mean starvation or consuming large amounts of liquids or certain types of products such as lemon in DASH diet to achieve weight loss.

CONS

In the initial phase, you will have to make an effort to change your eating habits;

Weight loss process is not very fast, but the weight loss achieved from this diet is highly stable and constant.

You need to spend more time in the kitchen because healthy food is always prepared independently in your own kitchen.

6

Recipes of DASH diet

Broccoli & sprouted green gram salad

Ingredients:

1 cup of steamed broccoli

½ cup of sprouted green gram

1 tbsp of basil

1 tbsp of lemon juice

Method:

Mix all of the ingredients in a bowl and mix them thoroughly.

Serve.

Smoked egg plant & kale salad with dates

Ingredients:

1 cup of smoked eggplant

1 cup of chopped kale leaves, fresh

½ cup of seedless dates

½ tbsp of oregano

Method:

In a bowl, add all of the ingredients except oregano.

Mix it thoroughly.

Add oregano and give a gentle mix.

Serve.

Chicken breast & kiwi salad

Ingredients:

1 cup of boiled chicken breast, shredded

1 cup of kiwi, cubed

1 tbsp of garlic powder

½ tbsp of black pepper powder

½ tbsp of almond milk

Method:

Mix all of the ingredients in a bowl.

Serve.

Broccoli with egg salad

Ingredients:

2 eggs, boiled

1 cup of broccoli boiled

1 tbsp of pepper powder

1 tbsp of lemon juice

½ tbsp of olive oil

Method:

In a bowl, add broccoli, lemon juice, pepper powder and olive oil.

Chop the eggs into small pieces.

Mix it with broccoli mix and serve.

Grilled chicken breast with mint dip

Ingredients:

1 whole breast

1 tbsp of thyme

1 tbsp of lemon juice

1 tbsp of olive oil

½ cup of mint leaves

2 tbsp of coconut milk

½ tbsp of lemon juice

Method:

In a bowl, add chicken breast and make impression with the help of fork.

Add lemon juice, thyme and olive oil to it.

Mix it.

Turn on the grille or oven with griller.

Grill at 2000C for 30 min.

In order to prepare mint dip, add mint leaves and coconut milk to the blender.

Blend thoroughly and add lemon juice to it.

Serve grilled chicken breast with mint dip.

Cucumber & beetroot salad

Ingredients:

1 cup of cucumber, sliced

½ cup of beetroot sliced

1 tbsp of lemon juice

Method:

In a bowl, add all of the ingredients and give a good mix.

Serve.

Sautéed chickpeas with mango dip

Ingredients:

1 cup of boiled chickpeas
¼ cup of onions, chopped
1 tbsp of chopped garlic
1 tbsp of Chinese chili
2 tbsp of chopped curry leaves
½ tbsp of grape seed oil
½ cup of mango
1 tbsp of thyme
½ tbsp of oregano
1 green chilli

Method:

In a blender, add mango, thyme, oregano and green chilli.

Blend into a smooth paste.

In a hot pan, add grape seed oil.

Add garlic, onions and sauté them.

Add curry leaves and boiled chickpeas.

Sauté them thoroughly.

Add chopped curry leaves and turn off the heat.

Serve with mango dip.

7

Motivation is the Secret

People are interested in increasing the chances of success in all areas of life. One of the best ways, is to have a positive mental attitude. A positive attitude does not bring only fortune, but a great health too. Is there a better fortune than a healthy body, mind and soul?

When we talk about positive mental attitude, we can receive it in many ways. But I would like to talk about the 07 most effective and simplest ways to get it going;

Focus on the present.

The worst problem of our life is that we worry too much about the future. Sometimes about decades forward. They can be your future plans, goals or dreams. But we do the same with our problems as well, most of the time. We think that the problems will increase. Even with small negative incidents we see our future getting ruined. The best ways to stop your pessimism is to focus on your present, and what you have and where you stand.

Use positive language

Do you count how many negative words you speak during a day? How many times do you complaint about your life, weather, work, studies and family?

It is important to understand that our words have a power. Our words always are in the shapes of our thoughts. Once we start speaking positive things, our thoughts start becoming positive. Once you replace your negative thought, your life becomes more interesting as positive things starts happening in your life.

Mix with positive people.

Even though many of us don't agree, there is an influence in our lives from the people around us. A negative set of people can make our life a hard one, while the positive people will make life more easy and interesting. Living a positive life has an effect on our health for sure. Our body reacts according to our mind and when we are pessimistic about things happening in our life depression, anxiety, hyperactivity occurs and we start losing appetite, lose weight or gain weight, sleeplessness and many others. This is not healthy at all. In the long run it can bring more serious disorders. Hence, think twice when you chose your close friends and family.

Remember that you are powerful.

Most of us want to be who others want us to be. But, that directly and indirectly can make you forget who you are what you are. Always learn to look at yourself the way you are. Accept the reality stop imitating and limiting yourself within the boarders which others create.

The stupidest thing we do is that, we let others label us saying he/ she is fat, thin, moody, stupid, lovely, miserable and etc. But, it doesn't mean that you should accept it. Make your own image to live yourself as a powerful you.

Be grateful

Instead of worrying about the past or the future, find some time to be grateful for all the things you have received in your life. Appreciate even the smallest things and these happy times. It will give you an encouragement to move forward in life.

Sometimes being grateful can also heal some wounds in your past .It also can teach you some lessons to handle the present problems. Above all, it can make you happy.

The DASH diet when in combination with this positive mental attitude, helps to achieve higher results than trying the diet alone. If you need to get plenty of benefits, you need to believe that you are going to get it. This positive mental attitude helps to keep up your spirit and enthusiasm to follow DASH diet.

8
Conclusion

As a conclusion, DASH diet is working way beyond its limitation and secures the body from harmful effects of obesity and its complications. Even though it is a special diet, but the actual basis of the diet lies in promoting balanced diet. In addition, DASH diet comes with benefits more than what it is designed for. This diet supplies the body with surplus amounts of nutrients and nurtures the body to regain its own health status. It is very important, that the DASH diet activates the body's self-healing mode and not only solve the today's problem, but also prevents the future problem.

Moreover, weight loss is the main goal, which is addressed by the DASH diet. At the same time, DASH diet also directly addresses the problems of high blood pressure or hypertension and prevents the complication that arises from obesity and hypertension.

Disclaimer

Introduction

By using this book, you accept this disclaimer in full.

No advice

The book contains information. The information is not advice, and should not be treated as such.

If you think you may be suffering from any medical condition you should seek immediate medical attention. You should never delay seeking medical advice, disregard medical advice, or discontinue medical treatment because of information in the book.

No representations or warranties

To the maximum extent permitted by applicable law and subject to section below, we exclude all representations, warranties, undertakings and guarantees relating to the book.

Without prejudice to the generality of the foregoing paragraph, we do not represent, warrant, undertake or guarantee:

- that the information in the book is correct, accurate, complete or non-misleading;
- that the use of the guidance in the book will lead to any particular outcome or result.

Limitations and exclusions of liability

The limitations and exclusions of liability set out in this section and elsewhere in this disclaimer: are subject to section 6 below; and govern all liabilities arising under the disclaimer or in relation to the book, including liabilities arising in contract, in tort (including negligence) and for breach of statutory duty.

We will not be liable to you in respect of any losses arising out of any event or events beyond our reasonable control.

We will not be liable to you in respect of any business losses, including without limitation loss of or damage to profits, income, revenue, use, production, anticipated savings, business, contracts, commercial opportunities or goodwill.

We will not be liable to you in respect of any loss or corruption of any data, database or software.

We will not be liable to you in respect of any special, indirect or consequential loss or damage.

Exceptions

Nothing in this disclaimer shall: limit or exclude our liability for death or personal injury resulting from negligence; limit or exclude our liability for fraud or fraudulent misrepresentation; limit any of our liabilities in any way that is not permitted under applicable law; or exclude any of our liabilities that may not be excluded under applicable law.

Severability

If a section of this disclaimer is determined by any court or other competent authority to be unlawful and/or unenforceable, the other sections of this disclaimer continue in effect.

If any unlawful and/or unenforceable section would be lawful or enforceable if part of it were deleted, that part will be deemed to be deleted, and the rest of the section will continue in effect.

Law and jurisdiction

This disclaimer will be governed by and construed in accordance with Swiss law, and any disputes relating to this disclaimer will be subject to the exclusive jurisdiction of the courts of Switzerland.

www.ingramcontent.com/pod-product-compliance
Ingram Content Group UK Ltd.
Pitfield, Milton Keynes, MK11 3LW, UK
UKHW042001190726
13854UKWH00005B/2107

9 798889 092667